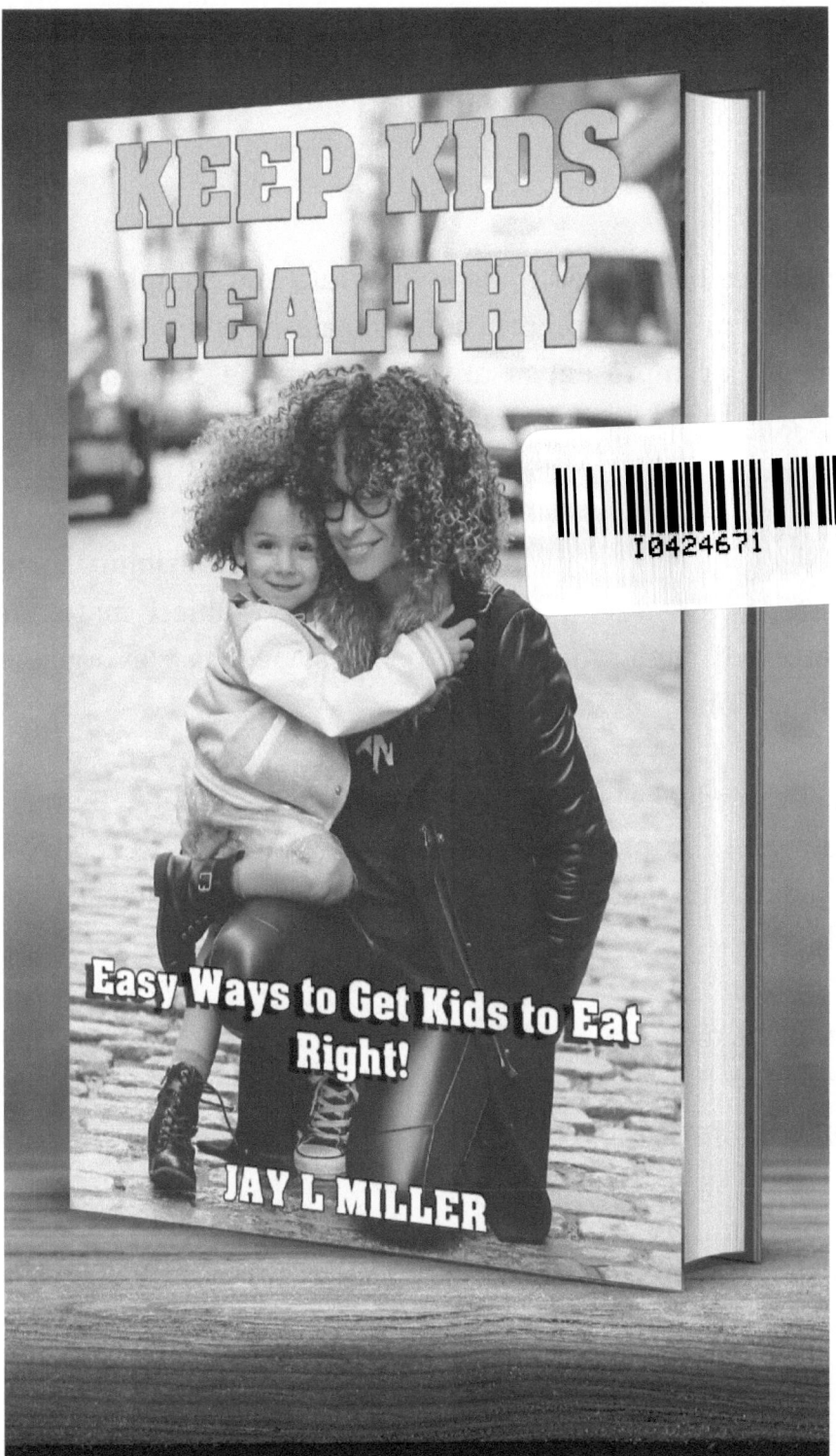

KEEP KIDS HEALTHY

Easy Ways to Get Kids to Eat Right!

JAY L MILLER

Terms and Conditions

LEGAL NOTICE

The Publisher has strived to be as accurate and complete as possible in the creation of this report, notwithstanding the fact that he does not warrant or represent at any time that the contents within are accurate due to the rapidly changing nature of the Internet.

While all attempts have been made to verify information provided in this publication, the Publisher assumes no responsibility for errors, omissions, or contrary interpretation of the subject matter herein. Any perceived slights of specific persons, peoples, or organizations are unintentional.

In practical advice books, like anything else in life, there are no guarantees of income made. Readers are cautioned to reply on their own judgment about their individual circumstances to act accordingly.

This book is not intended for use as a source of legal, business, accounting or financial advice. All readers are advised to seek services of competent professionals in legal, business, accounting and finance fields.

You are encouraged to print this book for easy reading.

Table Of Contents

Foreword

The need to ensure kids' health is one of the most important obligations of parents. In today's world where many adults tend to live with unhealthy and inactive lifestyle, it is crucial to teach your kids the essentials of health while they are still young. Get all the info you need here.

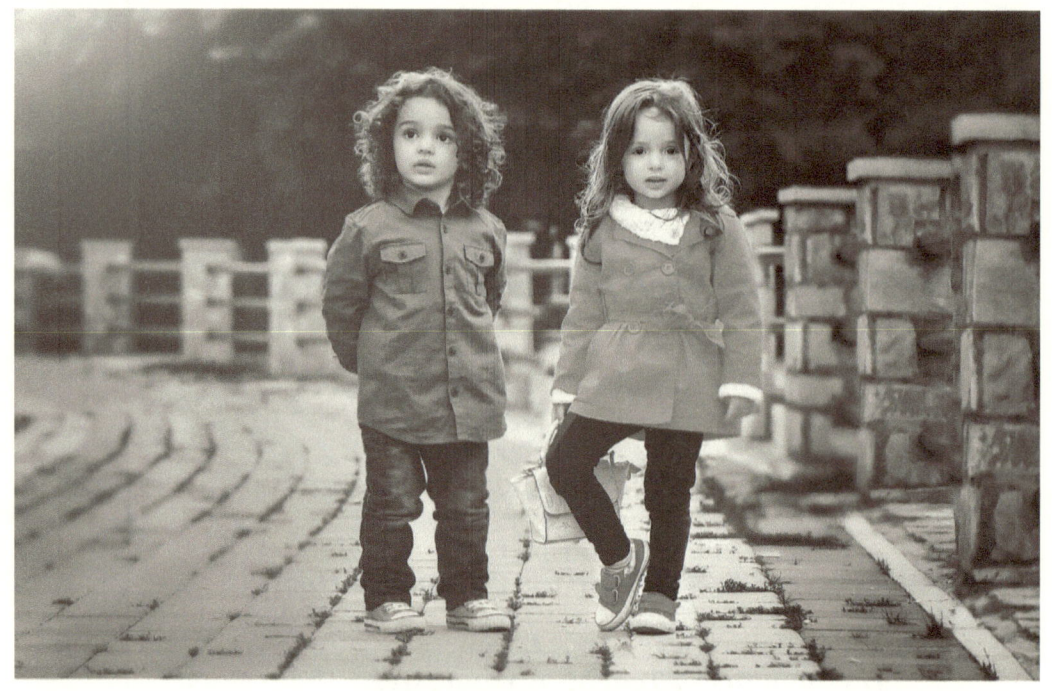

Healthy Kids

Everything You Need To Know To Give The Gift Of Health To Youngsters

Chapter 1:

Introduction

Synopsis

While you can still guide them, you need to help them understand the different aspects of their health. In doing this, you do not have to sound as if you are giving a sermon or a lecture. Through your nurturing and care along with their other daily activities, you can ensure that your kids have healthy and balanced lifestyle.

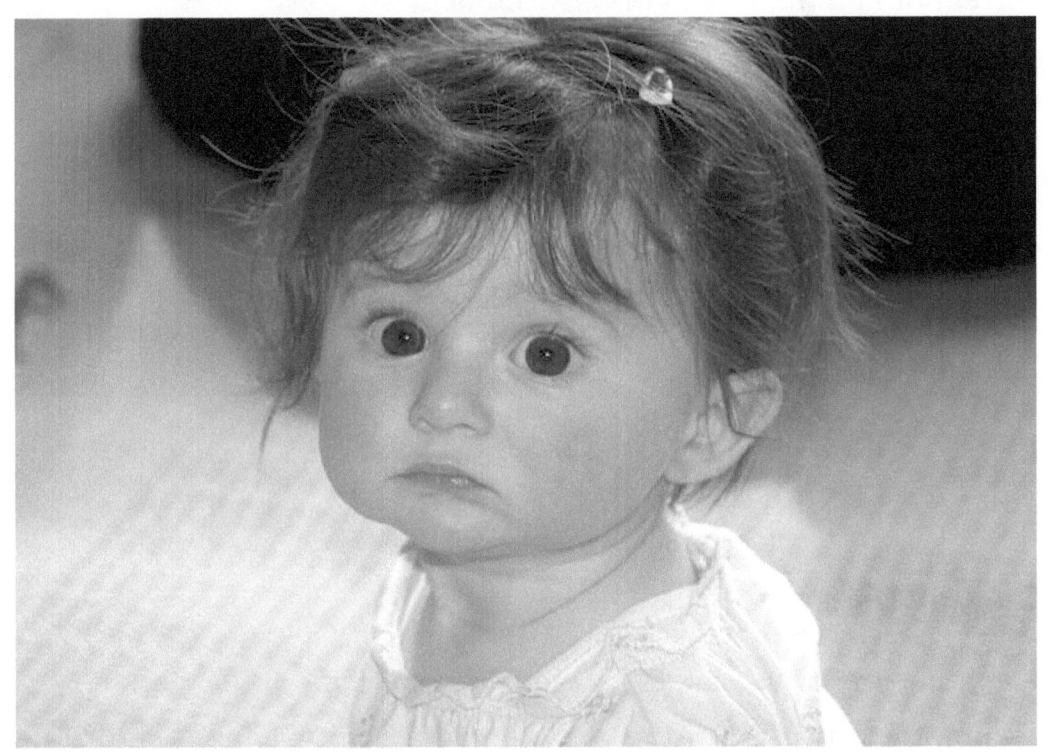

The Basics

Developing the Right Habits

The habits that kids would develop will surely be carried on through their adult years. While they are still young, it is every parent's duty to help them develop the right habits. Along with character development, you should also take into consideration the daily habits of your kids, for instance, the foods that they eat, their physical activities, their relationship with other people and even their perceptions on things and the environment.

Kids do not have ample knowledge about the world. Most of the time, they get easily enticed with foods or even with activities they think are fun and enjoyable without taking into consideration the negative effects.

In order to help them, you need to discipline your kids in such a way that they grow to become individuals who are responsible, health conscious and mature.

Healthy Diet

Many parents if not all will encounter problems when it comes to feeding their children. After all, even adults are having a hard time eating a healthy diet for the main reason that by doing so, they have to eat nutritious yet tasteless meals.

The appetite of kids can be highly sensitive. Young children would often be easily enticed to eat foods that contain too much oil like fried chicken, French fries, etc. Several kids cannot refuse to eat chocolates, candies and other products that contain too much sugar. There is really nothing wrong with this. But everything that is too much can also be dangerous. As a parent, you need to monitor the foods that your kids eat. There are ways for you to provide creative meals that are both delicious and nutritious.

Physical Activities

Apart from their daily eating habits, kids also need to exercise. Considering their age, you cannot compel them to exercise if they do not want to do so. In guise of sports or other activities that involve playing with other kids, you can ensure that your kids if physically active. Not only does he/she enjoy the company of other kids, your child also gets the chance to exercise without him/her knowing it.

Learn Many Tips from This EBook

This is basically the main purpose of this EBook, to provide a holistic approach and insightful tips to ensure your kids' good health. The EBook is divided in different chapters covering balanced diet, exercise and even stress. With these useful tips, recipes and other important information, you get the chance to get to know more about the different dimensions of your kid's health.

Chapter 2:

What Youngsters Need For A Healthy Diet

Synopsis

To ensure that your kids have a complete and well-balanced diet, you need to know the specific kinds of foods that they have to eat along with the right amount of vitamins and minerals they need.

Many parents possess the general knowledge when it comes to foods to eat and foods to avoid. But there is also a need to know the right serving to target the complete amount of vitamins and minerals needed by the body.

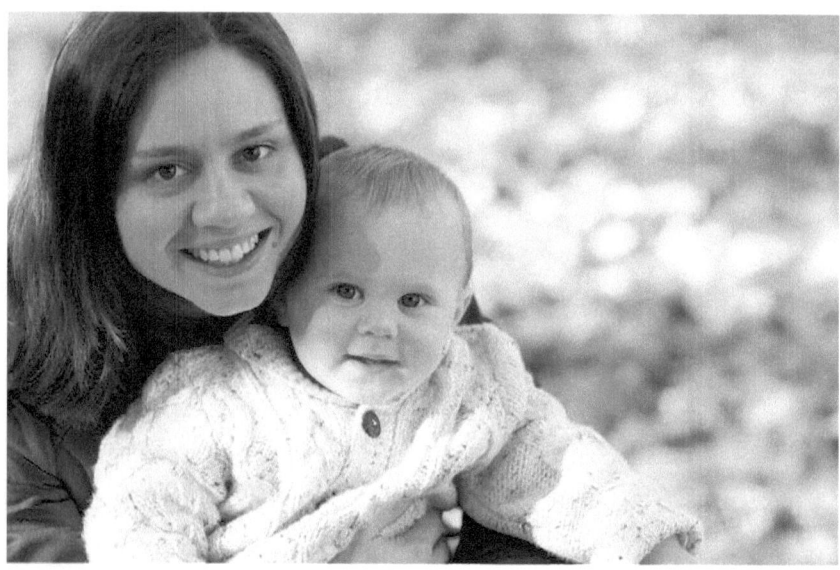

What Do They Need

Dietary Guidelines for Toddlers and Young Children

Toddlers and young children need to have the complete amount of nutrition for growth and development. As a parent, it helps if you know about the dietary guidelines so that you can prepare the right foods for them.

Whole grains: In the morning, you can have buckwheat pancakes or bread. At night, you can include brown rice for dinner. Just make sure that your kids get four daily servings of whole grains.

Fruits and Vegetables: Your kids need to have two servings of fruits and vegetables every day. In the morning, you can have apple or other snacks which contain fruits. You can also prepare soups using nutritional vegetables.

Protein: Kids need to have protein to develop their muscles. In a day, you need to have two servings. Encourage your kids to eat eggs, fish, lamb, chicken and baked beans.

Milk and Dairy: For your kid's bone development, you need to provide three servings. Your kid can have cheese, milk, yogurt, etc.

Vitamins and minerals: Using supplements can also help to ensure that your kids get the right amount of vitamins and minerals.

Nutritional Guidelines for School Age Children

As kids grow, they would require to eat more and to have the nutrition needed by adults. From eating whole grains (oats, rice, millet, etc.) to fruits, vegetables and healthy proteins, your kids also need to have healthy fats which include the following:

Monounsaturated fats: Avocados, canola oil, peanut oil, sesame seeds, etc.

Trans Fats: This type is found in crackers, cookies, margarines, etc.

Polyunsaturated fats: Omega 3 fatty acids (good for the heart) and Omega 6 fatty acids like salmon, sardines, anchovies, walnuts and a whole lot more.

Dietary Guidelines

Whole Grains: School age kids should have 6-11 servings of whole grains every day.

Fruits: For fruits, you should provide 2-4 servings in a day which may include ¾ cup of any fruit juice or ½ cup of sliced fruits.

Vegetables: 3- 5 servings are needed in a day. You can serve 3/5 cup of vegetable juice or one cup of leafy vegetables.

Dairy Products: 2-3 servings of yogurt, milk or natural cheese.

Zinc: To boost school performance and enhance memory capacity, it is essential to have zinc found in beef, pork, liver, milk, cocoa and poultry among many others.

Prepare Sumptuous and Nutritional Meals

Encouraging your kid to eat nutritional meals is a challenging task especially if your kid happens to have sensitive preference when it comes to food. To ensure complete vitamins and minerals, be creative with the meals that you prepare and always keep in mind that you should prepare delicious meals.

Chapter 3:

What Foods To Keep The Kids Away From

Synopsis

Kids just love sweets and other meals that lack nutritional value. Since the foods that your children take can definitely impact their growth and development, it essential to know which specific foods to avoid. Knowing which kinds of food products and meals to avoid can help you in guiding your kids when it comes to the food that they eat.

Of course, you cannot monitor your kids' activities 24/7 especially if they are in school. But while they are still young, you need to help them develop the right eating habits.

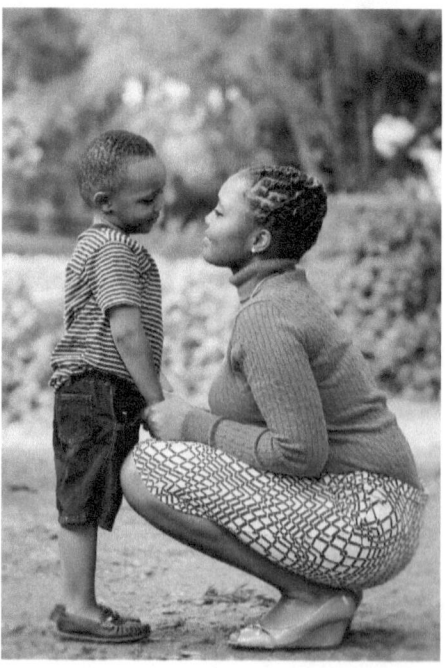

Stay Away From These

Limit Sugar

Everyone of use had our childhood experiences of eating different candies and chocolates. For children, they are at their happiest when they get to have these yummy candies and delicious chocolates. There is really nothing wrong in allowing your kids to have sweets. But you should make sure that they don't overdo it. According to the American Heart Association, children are limited to have 12 grams per day or 3 teaspoons a day.

There are ways for you to reduce sugar intake. For one, you can use less sugar whenever you prepare and cook meals. Another option is to avoid having sugary drinks like softdrinks and sodas. Instead of these drinks, you can replace nutritious smoothies. Lastly, you should not allow your kids to have processed foods.

Lessen Consumption of Products with Salt

Sodium is also needed for the body. But kids cannot have too much salt. One teaspoon of salt is already equivalent to 2,300 mg of sodium. There are guidelines when it comes to maximum salt intake recommended for young kids. For kids 1 to 3 years old, the maximum salt intake is 1,500 mg a day. Kids age 4 to 8 years old, they should not consume more than 1,900 mg of sodium in a day. For kids 9 to 13, the maximum salt intake is set at 2,200 mg per day.

How do you limit their salt intake?

There are several ways to lessen salt intake. Nowadays, many kids just love to go to restaurants and fast food. Most of these establishments make use of too much sodium. To lessen salt consumption, it is strongly suggested that you prepare meals at home instead of going to fast food restaurants.

It also recommended to have fresh vegetables instead of canned vegetables. When buying products, you must choose low salt products.

Avoid Eating Junk Foods

Junk foods are everywhere. For sure, your kids would also enjoy eating different junk foods. These products lack nutritional value and some of them even contain too much salt and sugar. As such, you need to encourage your kids to avoid eating junk food or if it is not possible, at least, they can lessen their junk food consumption.

There are different alternatives that are more nutritious. For instance, instead of having potato chips, your kids might as well have graham crackers, fruit dips, bagels, English muffins. Instead of having ice cream, your kids can enjoy frozen yogurt that has low fat or even fruit smoothies.

Chapter 4:

Easy Ways To Get Kids To Eat Right

Synopsis

Kids should have a healthy diet since they need certain vitamins and minerals to help them grow. With the right kind of diet, they can further develop their bodies, sharpen their minds and be more physically energetic and active.

Unfortunately, this is easier said than done as lots of parents have to deal different problems in this aspect. For one, youngsters are still to be guided as to which foods are healthy and which are not. Second, the natural tendency of most kids is to love eating foods that contain too much sugar like chocolates and candies. Third, it is part of their youth that they enjoy unhealthy foods like junk food and other oily food products.

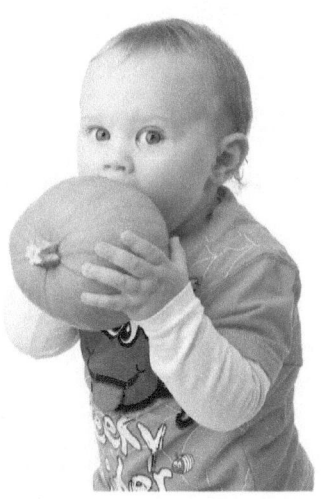

Do It The Easy Way

Develop the Right Eating Habits

It is important that you help them develop the right eating habits. You can still allow your kids to eat chocolates, fried chicken, etc. But you need to ensure that they eat more nutritional meals and that they get the complete vitamins and minerals needed by their body.

How do you exactly develop their eating habits?

- Have regular meals at home. Kids should know when it is the right time to eat and what meals to take. When you cook meals at home, you know the ingredients used are healthy used unlike if you will allow your kids to eat fastfood meals or buy food at the canteen. Prepare meals at home so you can easily monitor the foods that they eat.

- Allow them to participate. Kids also want to get involved. When you go to a supermarket, you can take along your kidz and allow them to select which items they can have for their lunch box. You should just monitor and sort out the items that they will choose and help them understand why they should avoid unhealthy food products.

- Prepare healthy yet nutritious meals. One of the main reasons why kids hate eating nutritious meals is that some would prepare meals that are not visually appealing and lack in taste. In order to attract your kids to eat healthy meals, you can search for certain recipes online in which you can prepare meals that have nutritional content without compromising the taste. Be creative when you prepare any meal. For instance, you might want to use some art techniques just to make a meal visually appealing.

- Encourage them to eat more fruits and vegetables. Every morning, you can prepare fresh and nice smoothies that your kids would surely love. Vegetables can also be used in different meals without them knowing it.

- Avoid serving meals in large portions. The number of kids suffering from obesity is increasing throughout these years. This can be a serious problem if neglected. To avoid having to experience this kind of problem, you should serve the right portion of every meal. If you notice that your kids tend to eat more than a normal kid would do then you should seriously consider in curbing their appetite to avoid gaining weight.

Chapter 5:

What Youngsters Need For Exercise

Synopsis

Just like adults, kids also need to exercise. Apart from just the importance of socializing and interacting with other people, kids develop their physical health whenever they exercise regularly.

Encouraging your kids to exercise is not that difficult since most kids enjoy playing and active. They like to run and have fun with other kids. These physical activities can already be considered as exercise.

Your kids can try different exercises and activities. Depending on their own preference, they can choose any activity that they want.

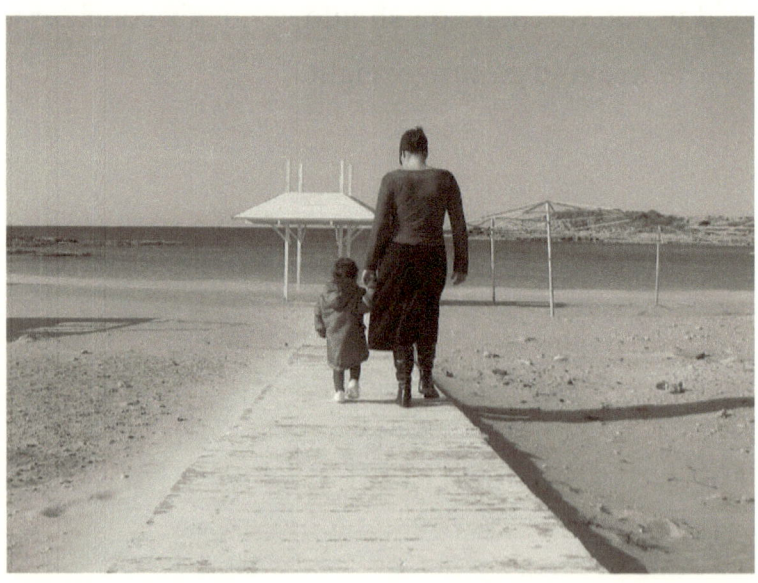

Exercise

Importance of Motivation

Most kids are active and the natural tendency is that they want to be playful most of the time. However, there are also kids whose personalities are quite different. Some would rather stay indoors and have activities that do not involve too many physical movements.

When this happens, the very first thing that youngsters need to exercise is motivation. This is also one of the most difficult things to do especially if kids are not interested at all. But with patience, parents can definitely find ways to motivate their kids to exercise.

Allotting Time for Exercise

When kids are busy in school and they have different activities that they need to do, it is important for parents to look after their daily schedules and make sure that there is a spare time allotted for exercise. By allotting one hour in a day, your kids can already exercise.

Sports and Other Physical Activities

Doing sports is one of the most effective kinds of exercise programs for your kids. Not only do they develop self-discipline but they also develop the over-all health of a person. You can either enroll your kid in a taekwondo class or other sports that he is interested in. Before he attends the class, you should purchase the necessary items that he needs including his taekwondo uniform.

For girls, you might want to enroll your kid in a skating class or in ballet school. Kids who are enrolled in a skating class need to have the right outfit as well as the ice skates. Kids who are in dance class needs dancing shoes. Having the right attire enables them to perform better and enjoy their classes.

The most important aspect that you should take into consideration whenever you choose any activity is your kid's interest. What are the things that they like to do?

Tools and Equipment

There are physical activities that might require certain tools and equipment. For instance, there are kids who want to try other sports like cycling, ice hockey and other activities that would require certain tools and equipment. Parents with children who are enthusiastic in these activities should definitely support them. Later on, these hobbies might develop and kids might start to develop their passion.

Parents really need to invest in their kids. Although you might have to shed out some money just to ensure that they work on their physical health, at least you get to provide for the needs of your kids. Of course, there are also other ways where children can exercise without having to spend that much.

Chapter 6:

Easy Ways To Get Kids To Exercise

Synopsis

Youngsters also need to exercise regularly to help them develop the different aspects of their health. Considering that vitality comes with a young age, children by nature are active and playful. As such, you will not encounter any difficulty in this aspect. When they run around and play with other kids, they already get the chance to exercise.

But on the other hand, there are also kids who are not that active. There are other kids who are quite timid and who are really not into physical activities. Some kids prefer to try other activity where they can't exercise.

If this is the case then parents should find ways to get kids to exercise. This can be a challenge if your child does not want to engage too much in physical activities.

Get Them Moving

How do you go about it?

1. Allow kids to socialize.

To get kids to exercise, you do not have to force them or to make them do the usual exercise programs done by adults. There are many kids who like to play in playgrounds and parks. Even if your kid is not physically active, he/she can still interact with other kids. By playing with his friends, it is already a form of exercise. Nothing beats the fun of running and playing around with other kids.

2. Encourage children to try sports.

Any sports activity is not just for adults. Even kids can try different kinds of sports depending on their preference. From swimming, taekwondo, table tennis to skating, they can just choose which particular sport they want to try.

There are several benefits that come along when kids are active in sports. For one, this is the best form of exercise especially when children try highly physical sports like swimming, judo, taekwondo and running among many others. Second, sports also help kids develop their sense of responsibility. They start to mature and they are more disciplined. Sports help in forming and developing the child's personality and character. This is primarily one of the reasons why there are so many parents who want to enroll their kids in different sports activities.

3. Parents should join their children to make physical activities more fun.

From time to time, parents can join their children in any physical activity that they do. When kids see their mom or dad playing with them, they are more motivated. Parents also get the chance to bond and spend quality time with their kids. Every weekend, you can plan different activities for your children and let them have fun. There are lots of things that you can share with your kids where they get the chance to exercise their bodies.

4. Try indoor activities.

For kids who really do not want to go out that much, there are indoor activities that they can try. There are gaming consoles where kids get to move and can exercise. Parents can also invest in different tools and equipment where kids can exercise even if they are at home.

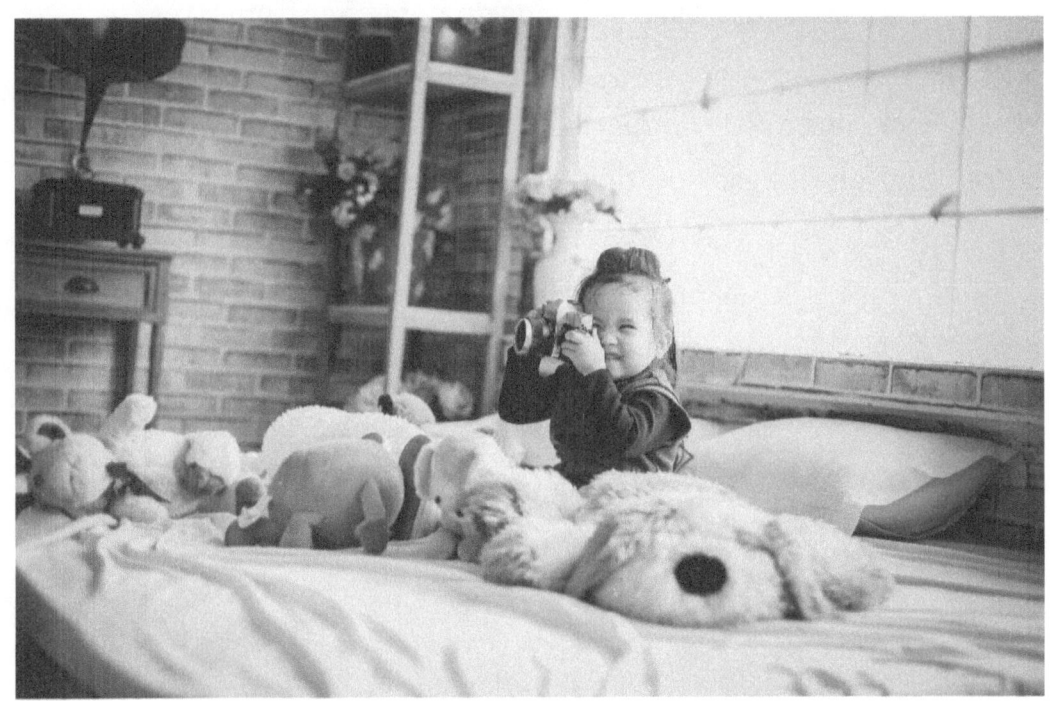

Chapter 7:

The Impact Stress Has On Kids

Synopsis

Stress is one of the leading factors why many people get certain diseases and illnesses. Although adults are more prone to experience stress due to work, kind of lifestyle and personal relationships, kids are also not immune. There are many factors that can contribute to stress. At home or even in schools, children can experience stress.

With the intricate relationships that people have these days and with the kind of environment that surround them, it is difficult to shield your kids from stressful situations. As such, parents must do their best in order to ensure that their kids do not suffer from stress.

Stress can negatively impact a kid's behavior and even their perceptions on things. How does stress affect kids?

Tension And Kids

1. Stress affects the mental development of kids.

Research would show that those kids who encounter stressful situations are more likely to experience problems in their mental development. When a kid is stressed out, challenges arise. At school, kids cannot concentrate on their studies. Their concentration can also be affected which can then affect their over-all performance in school.

2. Stress can drastically change the behavior of kids.

Youngsters who experience stress at home and in school would tend to suffer from drastic changes in behavior. One of the most evident results is that kids who suffer major stress would stay away from other people and are aloof. They tend to lack themselves and avoid socializing with other people.

Some kids who suffer from stressful situations may experience low self-esteem. This affects how they interact with other people and how they look at themselves.

3. Stress can affect their eating habits.

To ensure your kid's growth and development, you need to provide foods with complete nutrition. Aside from just providing healthy meals for them, you should also make sure that your kids do not experience stress at home. When a kid is stressed out, his eating habits may change. Some would tend to eat too much which can later on result to obesity while there are other kids who would lose their appetite and would not eat.

When this happens, their over-all growth and development will be highly affected. Without complete nutrition and with all the stress they have to go through, kids might experience health problems and other health risks associated with stress.

How Can Kids Avoid Stress?

Unlike adults who have to live and face the world on their own, kids are sheltered by their families and other loved ones. As innocent and young as they are, they should not be facing stressful situations that can negatively affect their attitude, behavior and even character in the long run.

As a parent, it is your obligation to make sure that your kids grow in a peaceful, secured and stress-free environment. Of course, stressful situations cannot be totally avoided. But as a parent, you should try your very best to shield and to protect your children while they are still young. After all, they do not know much about the complicated matters that surround them.

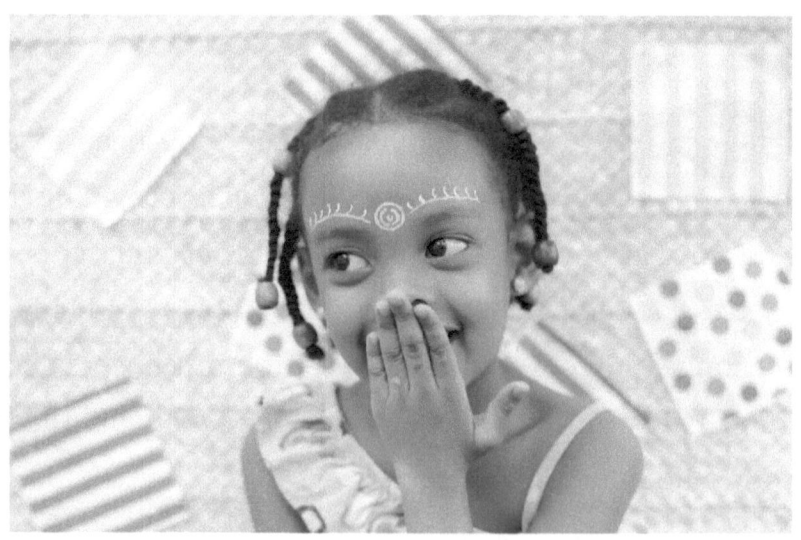

Chapter 8:

How To Help Youngsters De-stress

Synopsis

Youngsters at some point in their life may experience stress. This is something that parents and kids cannot avoid. For instance, when a kid sees his parents arguing or fighting, it can be really stressful. When kids experience problems in school, it can also lead to stress.

Parents cannot really avoid and fully protect their kids from stressful situations. But what parents can do is to find ways to help their kids de-stress. When a kid suffers from stress, it is important that he/she has a strong support group.

What are the different ways that you can do to help your kids de-stress?

How To Help

1. Importance of Communication

Many parents with their tight schedules and other obligations tend to forget the importance of communication. Although they attend to their kid's needs, some barely spend time to ask how their kids are doing in school or how they are coping. Without contact communication, kids might feel alone. When something bad happens or when they experience any stressful situation, they will definitely have a hard time in coping with the problem. They do not want to share it with other people.

That is why it is crucial that parents constantly communicate with their kids. When kids talk to their parents, they can share their thoughts and feelings. If they feel any stress, they do not have to carry the burden alone. Their parents can definitely comfort them.

2. Make Time for Your Kids

Family relations are also very important especially since youngsters have to face certain stages in growth and development where they may face tough situations that they find really stressful. As such, it is essential that kids do not feel as if they are alone in this journey.

Parents should always show their kids how much they love them and how much they care. No matter how busy you are, you should always look for ways to reach and connect to your kids. Even with your busy schedule, you should have spare time where you can bond with your kids and show them how important they are. When kids feel loved at home, they can overcome tough situations easily.

3. Ensure Good Health

To make your kids active and vibrant in school, you should make sure that you provide all of their needs especially in terms of their over-all health. Prepare meals that would boost their energy and hone their minds. Kids who eat nutritious meals and those who have the complete daily requirements of vitamins and minerals are less likely to suffer from stress.

Having complete sleep is also an important factor. When a child barely has enough sleep, the tendency is for him/her to get easily irritated. Make sure that your kids sleep early and that they have complete sleeping time.

4. Grace Under Pressure

Children tend to follow what they usually see. The behavior and attitude of their parents towards certain events or instances can influence how kids deal with dress. That is why whenever parents face stressful situations, it is a must that they handle any problem with grace.

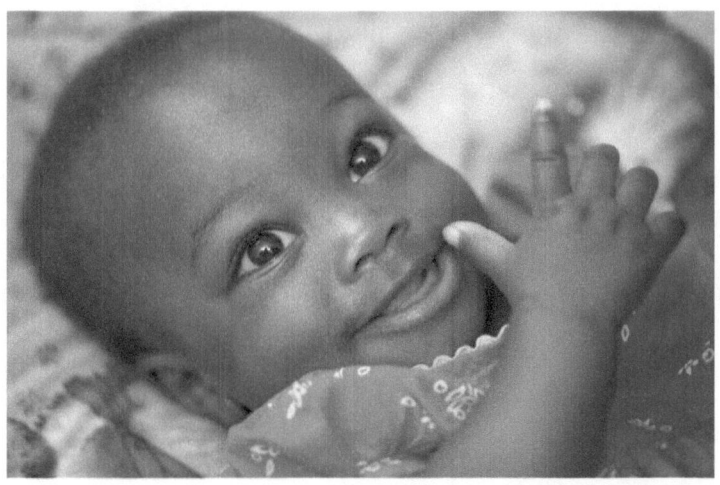

Chapter 9:

New Technology For Children's Health

Synopsis

Technology has brought significant changes not just for adults but even to children. When you go to different stores, you'll notice that there are a wide variety of modern products that your kids would surely love and enjoy. Apart from just the entertainment value that technology can give your child, there are also other aspects of your child's growth and development in which technology can be a good contributing factor.

In relating new technology and health, how can you make use of the available technology to improve your kids' over-all health? Is it really possible to use technology for children's health?

The answer is a definitely big Yes!

With the advancements of technology, there are now ways for you to develop the different aspects of your kids' health. These would include the following:

New Technology

Mental Health

One of the aspects that you can further develop with the use of technology is the mental health. Nowadays, many kids are more competitive and more intelligent. They can easily operate different kinds of gadgets and devices. For parents, it is now time to make use of the present technology.

For instance, parents who want to sharpen their kids' memory and to widen their imaginations can allow their kids to play different kinds of online games. Through a portable device, youngsters can enjoy several types of games where they get the chance to use their brains and think of certain strategies. Apart from that, they can also interact and socialize with other kids who are also playing the same game.

But of course, parents should still guide their kids whenever they spend time using these gadgets for education purposes.

Physical Health

Another aspect of health that you can work on with the use of technology is the physical health. With so many products available for kids, they can just choose which specific items they want to have in order to improve their physical health.

There are now gaming devices where kids get the chance to exercise and move their bodies. They can dance and play different sports without having to go outside since there are gaming devices which enable them to perform these functions. Not only do they get to enjoy but they can also exercise without them being aware they are actually doing an exercise.

Oral Health

Kids just love to eat sweets. From candies to chocolates, it is not that easy to control their appetite when it comes to sweets. Although parents can monitor the meals and food products that their children take, there are still cases where they just cannot possibly do it. The result is that some kids if not all suffer from major dental health problems. Some would experience tooth decay.

But thanks to technology, there are now several dental services along with the different dental treatment and procedures to ensure that your kids will have a complete set of white and shining teeth. Dentists now make use of the current technology to prevent any tooth decay and to help kids have good teeth.

Chapter 10:

The Benefits Of Teaching Youngsters About Good Health

Synopsis

At a very young age, you can already lay the foundations of ensuring the good health of your kids. Though they may not fully understand everything that you want to do, at least you get the chance to guide them. The foods that they eat can definitely impact their over-all growth and development.

As a parent, you can nurture your kids in such a way that you give them the right and complete nutrition and you provide a safe and healthy environment where they can grow. In teaching youngsters about good health, there are long term benefits.

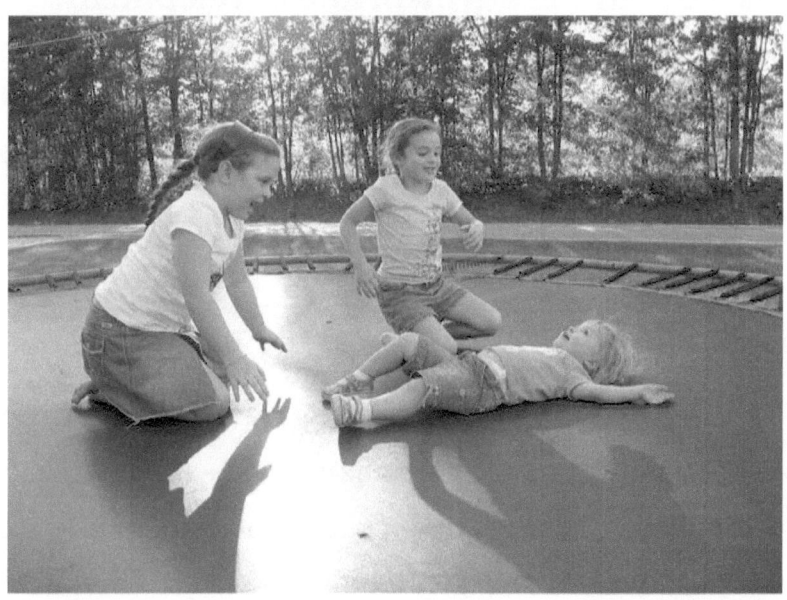

The Advantages

1. They develop the right habits.

A lot of adults who tend to have sedentary lifestyle usually have bad eating habits. Not only do they lack exercise but some would prefer to eat foods that contain too much fats, salt and sugar. Some would smoke or drink alcohol. All of these can be highly attributed to the kind of habits that they were able to develop when they were still young.

This is basically one of the reasons why it is important that while kids are still young, they start to form good habits. For instance, you should not allow your kids to consume foods that do not have nutritional content. When your kids prefer to eat vegetables and fruits, they will carry these good habits even when they get old.

2. You ensure your kid's growth and development.

Guiding your kid to develop the right habits is just one aspect. When parents teach their kids the importance of good health, they also ensure their kids development. The foods that kids eat may positively or negatively impact their growth. If parents allow kids to eat whatever they want without ensuring that they have the complete nutrients then this can negatively affect the growth of kids.

3. You lay the foundations and essentials of good health.

Aside from encouraging your kids to have good eating habits, you also lay the foundations of having good health. One evident example is that when your kid starts to become physically active in sports at an early stage, he/she can sustain that attitude later on. That is why it is strongly suggested that if kids love a particular sport, parents should really encourage their kids to participate in their chosen sports.

4. Kids can lessen stressful encounters.

When a kid has good health, he/she can avoid stress compare to other kids. Remember that the foods that your kids eat, their daily encounters and activities can add stress. But if your kid eats nutritional foods and they have regular exercises, he/she is expected to easily avoid stress.

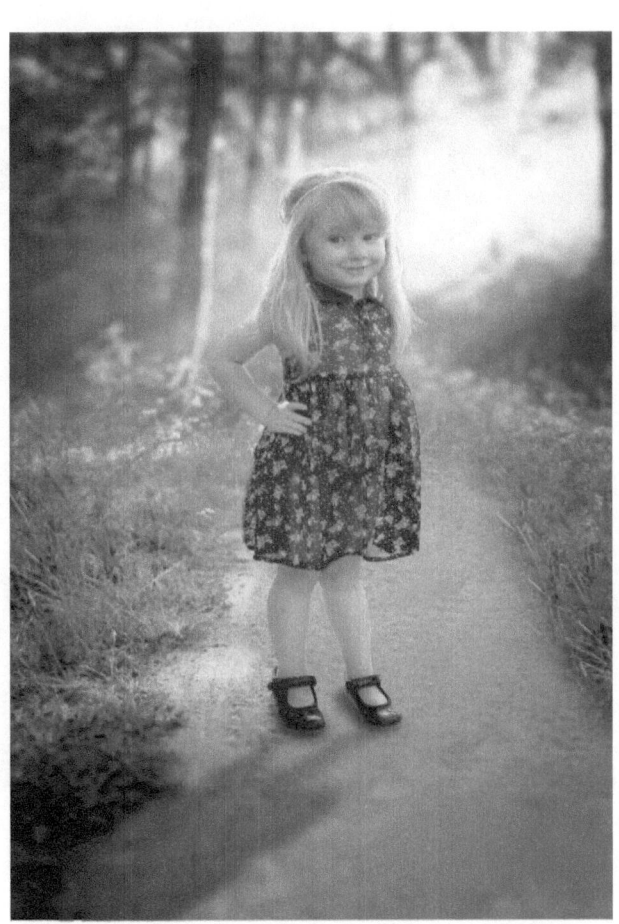

Wrapping Up

Helping your kid develop the right habits and lay the foundations of exploring the over-all health aspect can yield long term benefits. As a parent, it is your duty and obligation to provide the best kind of life that you can ever give. At least, when your kid grows and start to get older, he/she will always remember the things you taught.

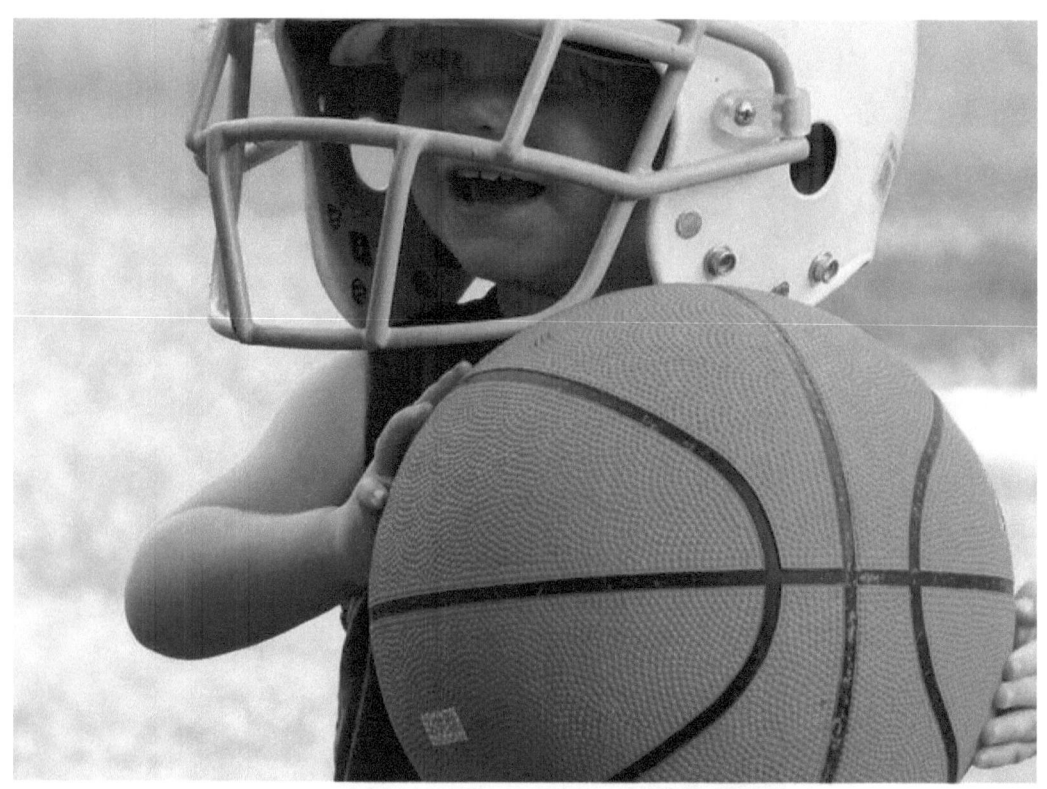